DR. BARBARA 7-DAY JUICE DETOX

Step-by-step guide to cleansing and rejuvenating your body and reviving your health using powerful, natural and nourishing recipes

Carlos Luz

Table of Contents

CHAPTER ONE 4

Introduction to Dr. Barbara's Herbal Juice Detox Program 4

Key Components of Dr. Barbara's Herbal Juice Detox Program 6

Benefits of Dr. Barbara's Herbal Juice Detox Program 7

Conclusion 8

CHAPTER TWO 8

Understanding the Benefits of Herbal Juicing for Detoxification 8

Detoxification and Its Importance..9

The Power of Herbal Juicing...9

Key Benefits of Herbal Juicing for Detoxification 10

Conclusion 11

CHAPTER THREE 12

The Science Behind Herbal Medicine and Detoxification 12

Understanding Herbal Medicine 13

Detoxification and Herbal Medicine..13

Scientific Evidence and Research..15

Conclusion 15

CHAPTER FOUR 16

Dr. Barbara's Principles of Herbal Healing and Nutrition 16

Conclusion 20

CHAPTER FIVE **21**

Preparing Your Body and Mind for the 7-Day Herbal Juice
Detox...**21**

CHAPTER SEVEN **28**

DR. BARBARA 7-DAY JUICE DETOX PLAN **28**

CHAPTER EIGHT..**35**

Herbal supplements and teas......................................**35**

CHAPTER NINE **39**

Managing detox symptoms...**39**

CHAPTER TEN **43**

Transitioning from a detox program back to solid foods **43**

BONUS: SOME HOLISTIC REMEDIES TO KNOW **47**

THE END...**84**

COPYRIGHT © 2023

CHAPTER ONE

Introduction to Dr. Barbara's Herbal Juice Detox Program

Dr. Barbara's Herbal Juice Detox Program is a holistic approach to cleansing and rejuvenating the body through the consumption of specially formulated herbal juices. Developed by Dr. Barbara, a renowned naturopathic with years of experience in herbal medicine and detoxification, this program aims to support the body's natural detoxification processes, promote overall health, and restore vitality.

Detoxification has been practiced for centuries in various cultures around the world as a means of purifying the body and eliminating toxins that accumulate from environmental pollutants, poor dietary choices, stress, and other factors. Dr. Barbara's Herbal Juice Detox Program builds upon this ancient tradition by incorporating modern scientific knowledge of herbs and their effects on the body's detoxification pathways.

The Science Behind Detoxification

Before delving into the specifics of Dr. Barbara's program, it's essential to understand the science behind detoxification. The body has its own built-in detoxification mechanisms primarily involving the liver, kidneys, skin, lungs, and lymphatic system.

These organs work together to eliminate toxins and waste products from the body, ensuring optimal health and functioning.

The liver plays a central role in detoxification by metabolizing and neutralizing toxins, making them easier for the body to eliminate. This process involves two main phases: Phase I, where toxins are converted into intermediate metabolites, and Phase II, where these metabolites are further processed and made water-soluble for excretion.

While the body's detoxification systems are highly efficient, they can become overwhelmed due to excessive toxin exposure or poor lifestyle habits. This is where detox programs like Dr. Barbara's Herbal Juice Detox come into play, providing additional support to enhance the body's natural detoxification processes.

Key Components of Dr. Barbara's Herbal Juice Detox Program

Dr. Barbara's program is based on the principles of herbal medicine, utilizing a combination of potent herbs known for their detoxifying properties. These herbs are carefully selected and blended to create powerful herbal juices that target different aspects of detoxification and support overall health.

One of the key components of the program is the use of organic, cold-pressed juices made from fresh fruits and vegetables. These juices are rich in vitamins, minerals, antioxidants, and phytonutrients that nourish the body and support detoxification. By consuming these nutrient-dense juices, participants provide their bodies with essential nutrients while giving the digestive system a break from processing solid foods.

In addition to the juices, Dr. Barbara's program may also include herbal supplements designed to further support detoxification and promote overall well-being. These supplements may contain a variety of herbs such as milk thistle, dandelion root, burdock root, turmeric, and ginger, all of which have been traditionally used for their detoxifying properties.

Benefits of Dr. Barbara's Herbal Juice Detox Program

Participants in Dr. Barbara's Herbal Juice Detox Program can expect to experience a wide range of benefits, both physical and mental. Some of the potential benefits include:

1. **Improved Digestion:** Giving the digestive system a break from solid foods allows it to rest and rejuvenate, leading to improved digestion and nutrient absorption.

2. **Increased Energy:** Many people report feeling more energized and alert during and after completing the detox program. This is often attributed to the elimination of toxins and the consumption of nutrient-dense juices.

3. **Weight Loss:** While weight loss is not the primary goal of the program, many participants may experience some degree of weight loss as a result of the detoxification process and the consumption of low-calorie, nutrient-dense juices.

4. **Clearer Skin:** Detoxifying the body can help eliminate toxins that contribute to skin issues such as acne, eczema, and dullness, leading to clearer, healthier-looking skin.

5. **Enhanced Mental Clarity:** Detox programs are often associated with improved mental clarity and focus. Many participants report feeling more mentally alert and focused after completing the program.

Conclusion

Dr. Barbara's Herbal Juice Detox Program offers a comprehensive and holistic approach to detoxification and overall health. By harnessing the power of herbs and organic juices, this program provides the body with essential nutrients while supporting its natural detoxification processes. Whether you're looking to jumpstart a healthier lifestyle, boost your energy levels, or simply give your body a much-needed reset, Dr. Barbara's program may be a valuable tool on your wellness journey.

CHAPTER TWO

Understanding the Benefits of Herbal Juicing for Detoxification

Herbal juicing for detoxification has gained significant popularity in recent years as people seek natural and holistic approaches to cleansing their bodies and improving their health. This practice involves consuming freshly made juices extracted from a variety of herbs, fruits, and vegetables known for their detoxifying properties. In this comprehensive exploration, we will delve into the myriad benefits of herbal juicing for detoxification, shedding light on the science behind this practice and its potential impact on overall well-being.

Detoxification and Its Importance

Before delving into the benefits of herbal juicing for detoxification, it's crucial to understand what detoxification entails and why it's essential for optimal health. Detoxification is the process by which the body eliminates toxins and harmful substances that accumulate as a result of environmental pollutants, dietary choices, stress, and other factors. These toxins can burden the body's organs and impair their functioning, leading to a wide range of health issues, including fatigue, digestive problems, skin disorders, and more.

The body has its own built-in detoxification mechanisms primarily involving the liver, kidneys, skin, lungs, and lymphatic system.

However, these systems can become overwhelmed by the constant onslaught of toxins in today's modern world. This is where herbal juicing comes into play, offering a natural and effective way to support the body's detoxification processes and promote overall health.

The Power of Herbal Juicing

Herbal juicing involves extracting the juices from various herbs, fruits, and vegetables using a juicer or blender. These juices are rich in vitamins, minerals, antioxidants, and phytonutrients that nourish the body and support detoxification. Unlike store-bought juices that may contain added sugars, preservatives, and other additives, freshly made herbal juices are pure and unadulterated, providing maximum nutritional benefit.

Key Benefits of Herbal Juicing for Detoxification

1. **Rich in Nutrients:** Herbal juices are packed with essential vitamins, minerals, and antioxidants that support overall health and well-being. These nutrients help nourish the body at a cellular level, providing the energy and vitality needed for optimal functioning.

2. **Hydration:** Proper hydration is essential for effective detoxification. Herbal juices are a hydrating and refreshing way to replenish fluids in the body, helping to flush out toxins and waste products through the kidneys and urinary system.

3. **Supports Liver Function:** The liver plays a central role in detoxification, metabolizing and neutralizing toxins for elimination. Certain herbs such as milk thistle, dandelion root, and burdock root have been traditionally used to support liver health and enhance its detoxification capabilities.

4. **Gentle on the Digestive System:** Herbal juices are easy to digest and require minimal processing by the digestive system. This allows the body to divert energy away from digestion and towards detoxification and repair processes.

5. **Alkalizing:** Many herbs, fruits, and vegetables used in herbal juicing have alkalizing properties, helping to balance the body's pH levels and reduce inflammation. An alkaline environment is conducive to detoxification and overall health.

6. **Promotes Weight Loss:** Herbal juicing can be an effective tool for weight loss as it provides essential nutrients while being low in calories. Additionally, the increased hydration and fiber content of herbal juices can help curb cravings and promote satiety.

7. **Enhances Skin Health:** The skin is a major detoxification organ, and herbal juices can help support its health and vitality. By eliminating toxins from the body, herbal juicing

can help improve skin complexion, reduce acne, and promote a youthful glow.

Conclusion

Herbal juicing for detoxification offers a myriad of benefits for overall health and well-being. By harnessing the power of herbs, fruits, and vegetables, herbal juices provide essential nutrients while supporting the body's natural detoxification processes. Whether you're looking to cleanse your body, boost your energy levels, or simply enhance your overall health, incorporating herbal juicing into your routine can be a valuable and enjoyable practice.

CHAPTER THREE

The Science Behind Herbal Medicine and Detoxification

Herbal medicine has been used for thousands of years as a natural and holistic approach to healing and wellness. With the rise in popularity of detoxification programs, there has been increasing interest in the science behind herbal medicine and its role in supporting the body's detoxification processes. In this comprehensive exploration, we will delve into the scientific principles underlying herbal medicine and its connection to detoxification, shedding light on how herbs can aid in the elimination of toxins and promote overall health.

Understanding Herbal Medicine

Herbal medicine, also known as botanical medicine or phytotherapy, involves the use of plants and plant extracts for medicinal purposes. Throughout history, various cultures around the world have developed their own systems of herbal medicine based on indigenous plants and traditional healing practices. Today, herbal medicine continues to be a valuable and widely utilized form of complementary and alternative medicine.

The therapeutic effects of herbs are attributed to their complex chemical composition, which includes a diverse array of phytochemicals such as alkaloids, flavonoids, terpenes, and phenolic compounds. These bioactive compounds interact with the body in various ways, exerting pharmacological effects that can help alleviate symptoms, support organ function, and promote overall well-being.

Detoxification and Herbal Medicine

Detoxification is the process by which the body eliminates toxins and harmful substances that accumulate from environmental pollutants, dietary choices, stress, and other factors. While the body has its own built-in detoxification mechanisms primarily involving the liver, kidneys, skin, lungs, and lymphatic system, herbal medicine can provide additional support to enhance these processes.

Certain herbs have been traditionally used for their detoxifying properties, helping to stimulate the body's natural detoxification pathways and facilitate the elimination of toxins. These herbs may exert their effects through various mechanisms, including:

1. **Liver Support:** The liver is the primary organ responsible for detoxification, metabolizing and neutralizing toxins for elimination. Herbs such as milk thistle, dandelion root, burdock root, and turmeric have been shown to support liver function and enhance its detoxification capabilities.

2. **Kidney Support:** The kidneys play a crucial role in filtering waste products and toxins from the blood, excreting them in the urine. Herbs like parsley, dandelion leaf, and nettle leaf

have diuretic properties that can help support kidney function and promote urine production.

3. **Antioxidant Activity:** Many herbs are rich in antioxidants, compounds that help neutralize harmful free radicals and protect the body from oxidative stress. Antioxidant-rich herbs such as green tea, ginger, and rosemary can help reduce inflammation and support overall detoxification.

4. **Lymphatic Drainage:** The lymphatic system plays a key role in removing toxins and waste products from the body. Herbs like cleavers, red clover, and echinacea have been traditionally used to support lymphatic drainage and circulation, aiding in the removal of toxins from the tissues.

Scientific Evidence and Research

While much of the evidence supporting the use of herbs for detoxification is based on traditional knowledge and anecdotal reports, there is also a growing body of scientific research that supports their efficacy. Studies have shown that certain herbs have hepatoprotective, nephroprotective, antioxidant, and anti-inflammatory properties, which can help support the body's detoxification processes.

For example, research has demonstrated that milk thistle extract, a popular herb used for liver support, contains active compounds such as silymarin that can protect liver cells from damage and promote regeneration. Similarly, studies have shown that dandelion root extract may have diuretic and liver-protective effects, making it beneficial for detoxification.

Conclusion

Herbal medicine offers a wealth of therapeutic potential for supporting detoxification and promoting overall health and well-being. By harnessing the natural healing properties of plants, herbal medicine can help stimulate the body's detoxification pathways, support organ function, and protect against oxidative stress and inflammation. Whether used alone or in conjunction with other detoxification strategies, herbs can be valuable allies in our quest for optimal health in a toxin-laden world.

CHAPTER FOUR

Dr. Barbara's Principles of Herbal Healing and Nutrition

Dr. Barbara's approach to herbal healing and nutrition is rooted in a deep understanding of the body's innate ability to heal itself and the therapeutic properties of herbs and whole foods. Through years of experience as a naturopathic doctor and herbalist, Dr. Barbara has developed a set of principles that guide her practice and empower individuals to take control of their health naturally. In this comprehensive exploration, we will delve into Dr. Barbara's principles of herbal healing and nutrition, shedding light on her holistic approach to wellness and the transformative power of plant-based medicine.

1. Holistic Healing Approach

Central to Dr. Barbara's philosophy is the belief in treating the whole person, not just the symptoms of disease. She recognizes that true healing involves addressing the underlying causes of illness and restoring balance to the body, mind, and spirit. This holistic approach considers all aspects of an individual's life, including their diet, lifestyle, environment, emotions, and spiritual well-being.

Dr. Barbara employs a variety of holistic healing modalities, including herbal medicine, nutrition, lifestyle counseling, stress management techniques, and energy medicine, to support the body's natural healing processes and promote optimal health.

2. The Power of Plants

Plants have been used for medicinal purposes since ancient times, and Dr. Barbara harnesses the healing power of herbs and botanicals to promote health and vitality. She believes that nature provides us with a vast pharmacy of healing plants that can support the body's innate ability to heal itself.

Dr. Barbara carefully selects herbs based on their traditional uses, scientific research, and individual patient needs, creating custom formulations to address specific health concerns. Whether it's supporting liver detoxification, balancing hormones, boosting immunity, or promoting relaxation, Dr. Barbara utilizes the therapeutic properties of plants to restore balance and harmony to the body.

3. Nutrient-Dense Whole Foods

Nutrition plays a crucial role in overall health and vitality, and Dr. Barbara emphasizes the importance of consuming nutrient-dense whole foods as the foundation of a healthy diet. She advocates for a plant-based diet rich in fruits, vegetables, whole grains, legumes, nuts, and seeds, which provide essential vitamins, minerals, antioxidants, and phytonutrients needed for optimal health.

Dr. Barbara encourages her patients to eat a rainbow of colorful fruits and vegetables to ensure they receive a wide variety of nutrients and phytochemicals. She also emphasizes the importance of organic, non-GMO, and locally sourced foods whenever possible to minimize exposure to pesticides, herbicides, and other harmful chemicals.

4. Individualized Care

Dr. Barbara recognizes that each person is unique and that there is no one-size-fits-all approach to health and wellness. She takes the time to listen to her patients' concerns, assess their individual health needs, and develop personalized treatment plans tailored to their specific goals and preferences.

Whether it's designing an herbal protocol, creating a customized nutrition plan, recommending lifestyle modifications, or providing emotional support, Dr. Barbara works collaboratively with her patients to empower them to take charge of their health and achieve their wellness goals.

5. Education and Empowerment

Education is a cornerstone of Dr. Barbara's practice, and she is committed to empowering her patients with the knowledge and tools they need to make informed decisions about their health. She provides comprehensive education on the benefits of herbal medicine, nutrition, lifestyle changes, and self-care practices, equipping her patients with the skills they need to maintain optimal health and prevent illness.

Dr. Barbara believes that true healing begins from within and that each person has the power to unlock their innate healing potential. By educating and empowering her patients, she helps them become active participants in their own health journey, leading to lasting transformations and improved quality of life.

Conclusion

Dr. Barbara's principles of herbal healing and nutrition offer a holistic approach to wellness that honors the body's innate ability to heal itself. Through the power of plants, nutrient-dense whole foods, individualized care, and education, Dr. Barbara empowers her patients to take control of their health naturally and achieve vibrant health and vitality. Her compassionate and personalized approach to healing creates a supportive environment where patients can thrive and experience profound transformations in their health and well-being.

CHAPTER FIVE

Preparing Your Body and Mind for the 7-Day Herbal Juice Detox

Embarking on a 7-day herbal juice detox can be a transformative experience for both your body and mind. However, proper preparation is essential to ensure a smooth and successful detoxification process. In this comprehensive guide, we will explore the steps you can take to prepare your body and mind for the 7-day herbal juice detox, setting the stage for a rejuvenating and revitalizing experience.

1. Consult with a Healthcare Professional

Before starting any detox program, it's important to consult with a qualified healthcare professional, especially if you have any underlying health conditions or are taking medications. They can provide personalized guidance and ensure that a detox program is safe and appropriate for you.

2. Set Clear Intentions

Setting clear intentions for your detox journey can help you stay focused and motivated throughout the process. Take some time to reflect on why you want to do the detox and what you hope to achieve. Whether it's to boost energy levels, support digestion, or kickstart healthy habits, clarifying your intentions can help keep you on track.

3. Gradually Transition to a Plant-Based Diet

In the days leading up to the detox, gradually transition to a plant-based diet rich in fruits, vegetables, whole grains, legumes, nuts, and seeds. This will help prepare your body for the detoxification process and minimize potential detox symptoms such as headaches, fatigue, and digestive issues.

4. Hydrate

Proper hydration is essential for effective detoxification, so be sure to drink plenty of water in the days leading up to the detox. Hydration helps flush toxins from the body and supports the functioning of your organs of elimination, such as the kidneys and liver.

5. Eliminate Processed Foods and Stimulants

Cutting out processed foods, caffeine, alcohol, and other stimulants can help reduce the toxic load on your body and prepare it for the detoxification process. These substances can interfere with detoxification pathways and may exacerbate detox symptoms, so it's best to avoid them during the pre-detox phase.

6. Stock Up on Supplies

Ensure you have all the supplies you need for the detox, including fresh organic fruits and vegetables, herbal teas, herbal supplements (if recommended), and any other ingredients specified in the detox program. Having everything on hand will make it easier to stick to the plan and avoid temptation.

7. Create a Supportive Environment

Create a supportive environment for your detox journey by removing temptations and distractions from your home. Clear out any unhealthy foods from your pantry and fridge, and surround yourself with nourishing, whole foods that will support your detox goals. Additionally, enlist the support of friends, family, or a detox buddy who can cheer you on and provide encouragement along the way.

8. Practice Self-Care

Lastly, take time to nurture yourself and practice self-care during the pre-detox phase. Engage in activities that promote relaxation and stress relief, such as meditation, yoga, deep breathing exercises, or spending time in nature. Getting plenty of rest and prioritizing sleep will also support your body's natural detoxification processes and set the stage for a successful detox experience.

By following these steps to prepare your body and mind for the 7-day herbal juice detox, you can maximize the benefits of the program and set yourself up for a transformative and rejuvenating experience. With proper preparation and a positive mindset, you'll be well-equipped to embark on your detox journey and emerge feeling refreshed, revitalized, and renewed.

CHAPTER SIX

Selecting the right herbs for detoxification and healing is essential to support your body's natural detoxification processes and promote overall health and well-being. With a myriad of herbs available, each possessing unique properties and benefits, it's important to choose the ones that best suit your individual needs and goals. In this guide, we'll explore how to select the right herbs for detoxification and healing, considering factors such as their therapeutic properties, safety, and compatibility with your health status.

1. Understand Your Goals

Before selecting herbs for detoxification and healing, it's essential to clarify your goals and intentions. Are you looking to support liver detoxification, improve digestion, boost immunity, or address specific health concerns such as inflammation or hormonal imbalance? Understanding your goals will help guide your herb selection process and ensure you choose herbs that align with your needs.

2. Research Therapeutic Properties

Different herbs possess varying therapeutic properties that can support detoxification and healing in different ways. For example, milk thistle is well-known for its liver-protective and detoxifying properties, while dandelion root stimulates bile production and supports liver function. Research the therapeutic properties of various herbs to identify those that are most relevant to your goals.

3. Consider Safety and Potential Interactions

Safety is paramount when selecting herbs for detoxification and healing, especially if you have underlying health conditions or are taking medications. Some herbs may interact with certain medications or exacerbate existing health issues, so it's essential to consult with a qualified healthcare professional before incorporating new herbs into your regimen. They can help ensure that the herbs you choose are safe and appropriate for your individual circumstances.

4. Choose High-Quality Herbs

Selecting high-quality herbs is crucial to ensure their potency and efficacy. Look for organic, non-GMO herbs from reputable sources that adhere to strict quality standards. Freshness and purity are key considerations when choosing herbs, so opt for herbs that have been sustainably harvested and processed using gentle extraction methods to preserve their beneficial compounds.

5. Customize Your Herbal Protocol

Every individual is unique, and what works for one person may not necessarily work for another. Customize your herbal protocol based on your specific needs, preferences, and health status. Consider factors such as dosage, frequency of use, and the method of administration (e.g., teas, tinctures, capsules) when designing your herbal regimen.

6. Start Slowly and Listen to Your Body

When incorporating new herbs into your routine, start slowly and gradually increase the dosage as needed. Pay attention to how your body responds to the herbs and listen to any signals or feedback it may provide. If you experience any adverse reactions or discomfort, discontinue use and consult with a healthcare professional.

7. Focus on Whole-Body Support

While targeting specific organs or systems for detoxification and healing is important, it's also essential to focus on whole-body support. Choose herbs that have a broad spectrum of benefits and support overall health and well-being, such as adaptogens that help the body adapt to stress or nutritive herbs that provide essential vitamins and minerals.

8. Incorporate Variety

Variety is key when it comes to herbal medicine, as different herbs offer unique benefits and therapeutic properties.

Incorporate a diverse range of herbs into your regimen to ensure comprehensive support for detoxification and healing. Experiment with different herbs and herbal combinations to find what works best for you.

By following these guidelines for selecting the right herbs for detoxification and healing, you can create a customized herbal protocol that supports your individual needs and goals. Whether you're looking to cleanse and rejuvenate your body, support specific organ function, or promote overall health and vitality, choosing the right herbs is an essential step towards achieving optimal wellness.

CHAPTER SEVEN

DR. BARBARA 7-DAY JUICE DETOX PLAN

Crafting herbal juice recipes for each day of your detox program can add variety, flavor, and therapeutic benefits to your cleansing journey. These recipes incorporate a blend of herbs, fruits, and vegetables known for their detoxifying properties, nourishing your body while supporting its natural detoxification processes. Below are seven herbal juice recipes—one for each day of your detox program—to help you feel refreshed, revitalized, and rejuvenated.

Day 1: Green Detox Elixir

Ingredients:

- 1 cucumber
- 2 celery stalks
- 1 green apple
- Handful of spinach
- 1 inch piece of ginger
- Handful of parsley
- Juice of 1 lemon

Instructions:

1. Wash all ingredients thoroughly.

2. Peel the cucumber if not organic, otherwise leave the skin on for added nutrients.

3. Core the apple and cut it into chunks.

4. Chop the celery stalks into smaller pieces.

5. Place all ingredients into a juicer and process until smooth.

6. Squeeze in the juice of one lemon and stir well.

7. Serve immediately and enjoy!

Day 2: Beet & Berry Cleanse

Ingredients:

- 1 medium beetroot

- 1 cup mixed berries (such as strawberries, blueberries, raspberries)

- 2 carrots

- 1-inch piece of turmeric root

- Handful of mint leaves

- Juice of 1 lime

Instructions:

1. Scrub the beetroot and carrots clean, then chop them into smaller pieces.

2. Rinse the berries and mint leaves under cold water.

3. Peel the turmeric root.

4. Add all ingredients to a juicer and blend until smooth.

5. Squeeze in the juice of one lime and mix well.

6. Pour into glasses and serve immediately.

Day 3: Citrus Cleanse Blast

Ingredients:

- 2 oranges

- 1 grapefruit

- 2 carrots

- 1-inch piece of ginger

- Handful of fresh cilantro

- Pinch of cayenne pepper (optional)

Instructions:

1. Peel the oranges and grapefruit, removing any seeds.

2. Scrub the carrots clean and chop them into smaller pieces.

3. Peel the ginger root.

4. Add all ingredients to a juicer and blend until well combined.

5. If desired, add a pinch of cayenne pepper for an extra kick.

6. Stir well, pour into glasses, and enjoy immediately.

Day 4: Pineapple Mint Detox Refresher

Ingredients:

- 2 cups fresh pineapple chunks

- Handful of mint leaves

- 1 cucumber

- 1 lime

- 1 inch piece of ginger

- 1 tablespoon of chia seeds (optional, for added fiber)

Instructions:

1. Peel and core the pineapple, then cut it into chunks.

2. Rinse the mint leaves and cucumber under cold water.

3. Peel the lime and ginger.

4. Place all ingredients into a juicer and blend until smooth.

5. If desired, add chia seeds for extra fiber and omega-3 fatty acids.

6. Stir well, pour into glasses, and serve immediately.

Day 5: Lemon Ginger Zinger

Ingredients:

- 2 lemons

- 1-inch piece of ginger

- 2 green apples

- Handful of kale leaves

- 1 cucumber

- Pinch of turmeric powder

Instructions:

1. Peel the lemons and ginger.

2. Core the apples and cut them into chunks.

3. Rinse the kale leaves and cucumber under cold water.

4. Add all ingredients to a juicer and blend until well combined.

5. Sprinkle in a pinch of turmeric powder for added anti-inflammatory benefits.

6. Stir well, pour into glasses, and enjoy immediately.

Day 6: Berry Beet Blast

Ingredients:

- 1 medium beetroot

- 1 cup mixed berries (such as strawberries, blueberries, raspberries)

- 1 orange

- Handful of spinach

- 1-inch piece of ginger

- Juice of 1 lemon

Instructions:

1. Scrub the beetroot clean and chop it into smaller pieces.

2. Rinse the berries and spinach under cold water.

3. Peel the orange and ginger.

4. Add all ingredients to a juicer and blend until smooth.

5. Squeeze in the juice of one lemon and mix well.

6. Pour into glasses and serve immediately.

Day 7: Turmeric Spice Detox Elixir

Ingredients:

- 1-inch piece of turmeric root

- 2 carrots

- 1 apple

- Handful of kale leaves

- 1 cucumber

- Juice of 1 lime

- Pinch of black pepper (to activate turmeric)

Instructions:

1. Peel the turmeric root and carrots.

2. Core the apple and cut it into chunks.

3. Rinse the kale leaves and cucumber under cold water.

4. Add all ingredients to a juicer and blend until well combined.

5. Squeeze in the juice of one lime and mix well.

6. Add a pinch of black pepper to activate the curcumin in turmeric.

7. Stir well, pour into glasses, and enjoy immediately.

These herbal juice recipes offer a delicious and nourishing way to support your body's natural detoxification processes and promote overall health and vitality. Incorporate them into your 7-day detox program for a refreshing and rejuvenating experience. Cheers to your health and well-being!

CHAPTER EIGHT

Herbal supplements and teas

Herbal supplements and teas can be valuable allies in enhancing detoxification by supporting the body's natural cleansing processes and promoting overall health and well-being. From liver support to immune-boosting properties, these herbal remedies offer a variety of benefits that can complement your detox regimen. Below are some herbal supplements and teas known for their detoxifying properties:

1. Milk Thistle

Milk thistle is perhaps one of the most well-known herbs for liver support and detoxification. Its active compound, silymarin, has antioxidant and anti-inflammatory properties that protect liver cells from damage and promote regeneration. Milk thistle supplements are commonly used to support liver health and aid in detoxification.

2. Dandelion Root

Dandelion root is another herb prized for its liver-detoxifying properties. It stimulates bile production, which helps the liver eliminate toxins more efficiently. Dandelion root supplements or teas can support liver function and promote detoxification.

3. Burdock Root

Burdock root is renowned for its blood-purifying properties and is often used in traditional herbal medicine to support detoxification. It helps eliminate toxins from the bloodstream and supports the liver and kidneys in their detoxification processes. Burdock root supplements or teas can be beneficial for overall detoxification.

4. Turmeric

Turmeric is a potent anti-inflammatory herb that supports detoxification by enhancing liver function and reducing inflammation throughout the body. Its active compound, curcumin, has antioxidant properties that help neutralize free radicals and support cellular health. Turmeric supplements or teas can be beneficial for overall detoxification and inflammation reduction.

5. Ginger

Ginger is known for its digestive and anti-inflammatory properties, making it a valuable herb for supporting detoxification. It stimulates digestion, aids in the elimination of toxins, and reduces inflammation in the digestive tract. Ginger supplements or teas can support digestion and overall detoxification.

6. Green Tea

Green tea is rich in antioxidants called catechins, which have been shown to support liver health and promote detoxification. It also contains compounds that help boost metabolism and promote fat burning, making it a valuable addition to a detox regimen. Green tea supplements or brewed tea can support overall detoxification and promote weight loss.

7. Nettle Leaf

Nettle leaf is a nutrient-rich herb that supports detoxification by promoting kidney function and elimination of waste products from the body. It is a natural diuretic, helping to flush out toxins and excess fluids from the body. Nettle leaf supplements or teas can support kidney health and detoxification.

8. Peppermint Tea

Peppermint tea is known for its soothing and digestive properties, making it a valuable addition to a detox regimen. It helps relieve bloating, gas, and indigestion, promoting healthy digestion and elimination of toxins. Peppermint tea can be enjoyed throughout the day as a refreshing and digestive-supportive beverage during your detox program.

When incorporating herbal supplements and teas into your detox regimen, it's essential to choose high-quality products from reputable sources. Consult with a qualified healthcare professional before starting any new supplement regimen, especially if you have underlying health conditions or are taking medications. They can provide personalized guidance and ensure that the herbs you choose are safe and appropriate for your individual needs. With the support of these herbal remedies, you can enhance your body's natural detoxification processes and promote optimal health and well-being.

CHAPTER NINE

Managing detox symptoms

Managing detox symptoms and supporting your body's natural processes are crucial aspects of a successful detoxification program. While detoxifying the body can lead to temporary discomfort as toxins are released and eliminated, there are several strategies you can employ to minimize symptoms and promote overall well-being. From staying hydrated to practicing self-care, here are some tips for managing detox symptoms and supporting your body's natural processes during a detox program:

1. Hydrate

Staying hydrated is essential for supporting the body's natural detoxification processes. Drink plenty of water throughout the day to help flush out toxins and keep your body hydrated. Herbal teas, coconut water, and infused water with lemon or cucumber are also excellent hydrating options.

2. Eat Nutrient-Dense Foods

Fuel your body with nutrient-dense foods that support detoxification and overall health. Focus on whole foods such as fruits, vegetables, whole grains, legumes, nuts, and seeds. These foods provide essential vitamins, minerals, antioxidants, and fiber that nourish your body and support detoxification.

3. Incorporate Herbal Supplements

Consider incorporating herbal supplements known for their detoxifying properties into your regimen. Milk thistle, dandelion root, burdock root, and turmeric are just a few examples of herbs that support liver health and aid in detoxification. Consult with a healthcare professional before starting any new supplement regimen.

4. Practice Deep Breathing

Deep breathing exercises can help reduce stress, promote relaxation, and support detoxification. Take slow, deep breaths in through your nose, hold for a few seconds, and then exhale slowly through your mouth. Repeat this process several times throughout the day to calm your mind and support your body's natural detoxification processes.

5. Engage in Gentle Exercise

Engaging in gentle exercise such as walking, yoga, or tai chi can help support circulation, lymphatic drainage, and the elimination of toxins from the body. Aim for at least 30 minutes of moderate exercise each day to promote overall well-being and support detoxification.

6. Practice Self-Care

Take time for self-care activities that promote relaxation and stress relief. Activities such as meditation, mindfulness, hot baths with Epsom salts, and body massage can help calm the nervous system, reduce stress levels, and support detoxification.

7. Get Plenty of Rest

Getting adequate rest is essential for supporting your body's natural detoxification processes. Aim for 7-9 hours of quality sleep each night to allow your body to repair and regenerate. Create a relaxing bedtime routine and prioritize sleep hygiene to ensure restful and rejuvenating sleep.

8. Listen to Your Body

Pay attention to how your body is feeling and listen to any signals or feedback it may provide. If you experience detox symptoms such as headaches, fatigue, digestive issues, or mood changes, take it as a sign that your body is releasing toxins and adjusting to the detox program. Be patient and gentle with yourself during this process.

9. Seek Professional Guidance

If you're experiencing severe or prolonged detox symptoms, or if you have any concerns about your detox program, seek guidance from a qualified healthcare professional. They can provide personalized advice, address any underlying health issues, and help ensure that your detox program is safe and effective for you.

By incorporating these strategies into your detox program, you can effectively manage detox symptoms and support your body's natural detoxification processes. Remember to listen to your body, prioritize self-care, and seek professional guidance if needed. With the right approach, you can experience the benefits of detoxification and promote overall health and well-being.

CHAPTER TEN

Transitioning from a detox program back to solid foods

Transitioning from a detox program back to solid foods is a crucial phase of the process to ensure that you maintain the results you've achieved and continue to support your body's natural detoxification processes. Gradually reintroducing solid foods can help prevent digestive discomfort, support nutrient absorption, and ease your body back into a regular eating routine. Here's a guide on how to smoothly transition from a detox program to solid foods while maintaining your results:

1. Start Slowly

After completing your detox program, it's essential to reintroduce solid foods gradually. Begin with simple, easily digestible foods such as steamed vegetables, cooked grains (like quinoa or brown rice), soups, and broths. These foods are gentle on the digestive system and help ease your body back into a regular eating routine.

2. Focus on Whole Foods

As you reintroduce solid foods, prioritize whole, nutrient-dense foods that support your overall health and well-being. Include a variety of fruits, vegetables, whole grains, legumes, nuts, seeds, and lean proteins in your meals to provide essential vitamins, minerals, antioxidants, and fiber.

3. Chew Thoroughly

Take the time to chew your food thoroughly and mindfully, allowing your digestive system to properly break down and absorb nutrients. Chewing your food well can help prevent digestive discomfort and promote optimal digestion and nutrient absorption.

4. Pay Attention to Hunger and Fullness Cues

Listen to your body's hunger and fullness cues as you reintroduce solid foods. Eat when you're hungry and stop when you're satisfied, avoiding overeating or undereating. Tuning into your body's signals can help you maintain a healthy relationship with food and support your body's natural detoxification processes.

5. Stay Hydrated

Continue to prioritize hydration by drinking plenty of water throughout the day. Adequate hydration supports detoxification, promotes healthy digestion, and helps maintain overall health and well-being. Aim to drink at least 8-10 glasses of water daily, or more if needed based on your individual needs and activity level.

6. Incorporate Digestive Support

Consider incorporating foods and supplements that support digestion into your post-detox transition. Probiotic-rich foods such as yogurt, kefir, sauerkraut, and kombucha can help replenish beneficial gut bacteria and support digestive health. Digestive enzymes and herbal teas such as ginger or peppermint can also aid in digestion and alleviate digestive discomfort.

7. Listen to Your Body

Pay attention to how your body responds to different foods as you reintroduce them into your diet. Notice any changes in energy levels, digestion, mood, or overall well-being, and adjust your food choices accordingly. Your body's feedback can help guide you in making nourishing choices that support your health and vitality.

8. Maintain a Balanced Diet

Focus on maintaining a balanced diet that includes a variety of nutrient-dense foods from all food groups. Incorporate plenty of fruits, vegetables, whole grains, lean proteins, and healthy fats into your meals to ensure you're meeting your nutritional needs and supporting your body's detoxification processes.

9. Practice Mindful Eating

Engage in mindful eating practices to cultivate a deeper connection with your food and promote healthy eating habits. Pay attention to the flavors, textures, and sensations of each bite, and savor the experience of nourishing your body with wholesome, nutritious foods.

10. Continue Healthy Habits

Finally, continue to prioritize healthy habits such as regular exercise, stress management, adequate sleep, and self-care practices to support your overall health and well-being. These habits complement your dietary choices and contribute to a balanced and sustainable lifestyle.

By following these tips for transitioning from a detox program to solid foods and maintaining your results, you can continue to support your body's natural detoxification processes and promote long-term health and vitality. Remember to listen to your body, honor your hunger and fullness cues, and make nourishing choices that support your overall well-being.

Tila:

Definition: Tila, also known as linden flower or lime blossom, refers to the flowers of the Tilia genus, primarily Tilia europaea and Tilia cordata. These trees are native to Europe, but they are also cultivated in other regions for their fragrant and medicinal flowers.

Ingredients: Tila flowers contain various bioactive compounds, including flavonoids, phenolic acids, and volatile oils. These compounds are believed to contribute to the herb's medicinal properties, including its potential as a mild sedative, anxiolytic, and anti-inflammatory agent.

How to Prepare: Tila flowers are typically prepared and consumed as an herbal tea or infusion. To make tea, dried tila flowers are steeped in hot water for several minutes before being strained and consumed.

Dosage: The appropriate dosage of tila can vary depending on factors such as age, health status, and the specific preparation being used. It's important to follow the recommended dosage on the product label or consult with a qualified herbalist or healthcare professional for personalized guidance.

How to Use: Tila tea is typically taken orally. It's often consumed in the evening as a calming bedtime beverage or during times of stress or anxiety. It's important to use tila products as directed and to discontinue use if any adverse effects occur.

Side Effects: Tila is generally considered safe for most people when used in moderate amounts. However, some individuals may experience allergic reactions or digestive upset. It may also interact with certain medications or have adverse effects in individuals with certain health conditions. It's important to use tila under the guidance of a healthcare professional and to discontinue use if any adverse effects occur.

Valerian:

Definition: Valerian, scientifically known as Valeriana officinalis, is a perennial flowering plant native to Europe and Asia. It has been used for centuries in traditional medicine for its potential calming and sedative effects.

Ingredients: Valerian root contains several bioactive compounds, including valerenic acid, valepotriates, and volatile oils. These compounds are believed to contribute to the herb's medicinal properties, including its potential as a sedative, anxiolytic, and sleep aid.

How to Prepare: Valerian root is typically prepared and consumed as an herbal tea, tincture, or capsule. To make tea, dried valerian root is steeped in hot water for several minutes before being strained and consumed. Tinctures are prepared by steeping the root in alcohol or vinegar to extract its active compounds.

Dosage: The appropriate dosage of valerian can vary depending on factors such as age, health status, and the specific preparation being used. It's important to follow the recommended dosage on the product label or consult with a qualified herbalist or healthcare professional for personalized guidance.

How to Use: Valerian tea, tincture, or capsules are typically taken orally. It's often consumed in the evening as a sleep aid or during times of stress or anxiety. It's important to use valerian products as directed and to discontinue use if any adverse effects occur.

Side Effects: Valerian is generally considered safe for most people when used in moderate amounts. However, some individuals may experience mild side effects such as drowsiness, headache, or gastrointestinal upset. It may also interact with certain medications or have adverse effects in individuals with certain health conditions. It's important to use valerian under the guidance of a healthcare professional and to discontinue use if any adverse effects occur.

Tila:

Definition: Tila, also known as linden flower or lime blossom, refers to the flowers of the Tilia genus, primarily Tilia europaea and Tilia cordata. These trees are native to Europe, but they are also cultivated in other regions for their fragrant and medicinal flowers.

Ingredients: Tila flowers contain various bioactive compounds, including flavonoids, phenolic acids, and volatile oils. These compounds are believed to contribute to the herb's medicinal properties, including its potential as a mild sedative, anxiolytic, and anti-inflammatory agent.

How to Prepare: Tila flowers are typically prepared and consumed as an herbal tea or infusion. To make tea, dried tila flowers are steeped in hot water for several minutes before being strained and consumed.

Dosage: The appropriate dosage of tila can vary depending on factors such as age, health status, and the specific preparation being used. It's important to follow the recommended dosage on the product label or consult with a qualified herbalist or healthcare professional for personalized guidance.

How to Use: Tila tea is typically taken orally. It's often consumed in the evening as a calming bedtime beverage or during times of stress or anxiety. It's important to use tila products as directed and to discontinue use if any adverse effects occur.

Side Effects: Tila is generally considered safe for most people when used in moderate amounts. However, some individuals may experience allergic reactions or digestive upset. It may also interact with certain medications or have adverse effects in individuals with certain health conditions. It's important to use tila under the guidance of a healthcare professional and to discontinue use if any adverse effects occur.

Valerian:

Definition: Valerian, scientifically known as Valeriana officinalis, is a perennial flowering plant native to Europe and Asia. It has been used for centuries in traditional medicine for its potential calming and sedative effects.

Ingredients: Valerian root contains several bioactive compounds, including valerenic acid, valepotriates, and volatile oils. These compounds are believed to contribute to the herb's medicinal properties, including its potential as a sedative, anxiolytic, and sleep aid.

How to Prepare: Valerian root is typically prepared and consumed as an herbal tea, tincture, or capsule. To make tea, dried valerian root is steeped in hot water for several minutes before being strained and consumed. Tinctures are prepared by steeping the root in alcohol or vinegar to extract its active compounds.

Dosage: The appropriate dosage of valerian can vary depending on factors such as age, health status, and the specific preparation being used. It's important to follow the recommended dosage on the product label or consult with a qualified herbalist or healthcare professional for personalized guidance.

How to Use: Valerian tea, tincture, or capsules are typically taken orally. It's often consumed in the evening as a sleep aid or during times of stress or anxiety. It's important to use valerian products as directed and to discontinue use if any adverse effects occur.

Side Effects: Valerian is generally considered safe for most people when used in moderate amounts. However, some individuals may experience mild side effects such as drowsiness, headache, or gastrointestinal upset. It may also interact with certain medications or have adverse effects in individuals with certain health conditions. It's important to use valerian under the guidance of a healthcare professional and to discontinue use if any adverse effects occur.

Wild Cherry Bark:

Definition: Wild cherry bark, scientifically known as Prunus serotina, is the bark obtained from the black cherry tree native to North America. It has been used traditionally in Native American and folk medicine for its potential health benefits, particularly for respiratory and digestive issues.

Ingredients: Wild cherry bark contains various bioactive compounds, including cyanogenic glycosides (such as prunasin and amygdalin), flavonoids, and phenolic acids. These compounds are believed to contribute to the herb's medicinal properties, including its potential as an expectorant, cough suppressant, and mild sedative.

How to Prepare: Wild cherry bark is typically prepared and consumed as an herbal tea, decoction, or syrup. To make tea, dried wild cherry bark is steeped in hot water for several minutes before being strained and consumed. Decoctions involve boiling the bark in water to extract its active compounds, while syrups are made by simmering the bark with sugar or honey to create a thick, sweet liquid.

Dosage: The appropriate dosage of wild cherry bark can vary depending on factors such as age, health status, and the specific preparation being used. It's important to follow the recommended dosage on the product label or consult with a qualified herbalist or healthcare professional for personalized guidance.

How to Use: Wild cherry bark tea, decoction, or syrup is typically taken orally. It's often consumed to soothe coughs, sore throats, and other respiratory symptoms. It's important to use wild cherry bark products as directed and to discontinue use if any adverse effects occur.

Side Effects: Wild cherry bark is generally considered safe for most people when used in moderate amounts. However, it contains cyanogenic glycosides, which can release cyanide in the body when metabolized. While the risk of cyanide poisoning from consuming wild cherry bark is low when used appropriately, excessive intake or prolonged use may lead to adverse effects. It's important to use wild cherry bark under the guidance of a healthcare professional and to discontinue use if any adverse effects occur.

Yellowdock:

Definition: Yellowdock, scientifically known as Rumex crispus, is a perennial flowering plant native to Europe and western Asia but is also found in North America. It has a long history of use in traditional medicine, particularly among Indigenous peoples, for its potential health benefits.

Ingredients: Yellowdock root contains various bioactive compounds, including anthraquinone glycosides (such as emodin and chrysophanol), tannins, and vitamins (including vitamin A and vitamin C). These compounds are believed to contribute to the herb's medicinal properties, including its potential as a laxative, blood cleanser, and liver tonic.

How to Prepare: Yellowdock root is typically prepared and consumed as an herbal tea, tincture, or capsule. To make tea, dried yellowdock root is steeped in hot water for several minutes before being strained and consumed. Tinctures are prepared by steeping the root in alcohol or vinegar to extract its active compounds.

Dosage: The appropriate dosage of yellowdock can vary depending on factors such as age, health status, and the specific preparation being used. It's important to follow the recommended dosage on the product label or consult with a qualified herbalist or healthcare professional for personalized guidance.

How to Use: Yellowdock tea, tincture, or capsules are typically taken orally. It's often consumed to support digestion, promote bowel regularity, and cleanse the blood. It's important to use yellowdock products as directed and to discontinue use if any adverse effects occur.

Side Effects: Yellowdock is generally considered safe for most people when used in moderate amounts. However, some individuals may experience mild side effects such as gastrointestinal upset or allergic reactions. It may also interact with certain medications or have adverse effects in individuals with certain health conditions. It's important to use yellowdock under the guidance of a healthcare professional and to discontinue use if any adverse effects occur.

Yellowdock Root:

Definition: Yellowdock root, scientifically known as Rumex crispus, is the root of a perennial flowering plant native to Europe and western Asia, also found in North America. It has a long history of use in traditional medicine, particularly among Indigenous peoples, for its potential health benefits.

Ingredients: Yellowdock root contains various bioactive compounds, including anthraquinone glycosides (such as emodin and chrysophanol), tannins, and vitamins (including vitamin A and vitamin C). These compounds are believed to contribute to the herb's medicinal properties, including its potential as a laxative, blood cleanser, and liver tonic.

How to Prepare: Yellowdock root is typically prepared and consumed as an herbal tea, tincture, or capsule. To make tea, dried yellowdock root is steeped in hot water for several minutes before being strained and consumed. Tinctures are prepared by steeping the root in alcohol or vinegar to extract its active compounds.

Dosage: The appropriate dosage of yellowdock root can vary depending on factors such as age, health status, and the specific preparation being used. It's important to follow the recommended dosage on the product label or consult with a qualified herbalist or healthcare professional for personalized guidance.

How to Use: Yellowdock root tea, tincture, or capsules are typically taken orally. It's often consumed to support digestion, promote bowel regularity, and cleanse the blood. It's important to use yellowdock root products as directed and to discontinue use if any adverse effects occur.

Side Effects: Yellowdock root is generally considered safe for most people when used in moderate amounts. However, some individuals may experience mild side effects such as gastrointestinal upset or allergic reactions. It may also interact with certain medications or have adverse effects in individuals with certain health conditions. It's important to use yellowdock root under the guidance of a healthcare professional and to discontinue use if any adverse effects occur.

Agrimony:

Definition: Agrimony, scientifically known as Agrimonia eupatoria, is a perennial herbaceous plant native to Europe, Asia, and North America. It has a long history of use in traditional medicine, particularly in European folk medicine, for its potential health benefits.

Ingredients: Agrimony contains various bioactive compounds, including tannins, flavonoids, phenolic acids, and volatile oils. These compounds are believed to contribute to the herb's medicinal properties, including its potential as an astringent, anti-inflammatory, and digestive aid.

How to Prepare: Agrimony is typically prepared and consumed as an herbal tea, tincture, or poultice. To make tea, dried agrimony leaves and flowers are steeped in hot water for several minutes before being strained and consumed. Tinctures are prepared by steeping the herb in alcohol or vinegar to extract its active compounds.

Dosage: The appropriate dosage of agrimony can vary depending on factors such as age, health status, and the specific preparation being used. It's important to follow the recommended dosage on the product label or consult with a qualified herbalist or healthcare professional for personalized guidance.

How to Use: Agrimony tea, tincture, or poultice is typically taken orally or applied topically. It's often consumed to soothe gastrointestinal issues, such as indigestion and diarrhea, or used externally to treat skin conditions.

Side Effects: Agrimony is generally considered safe for most people when used in moderate amounts. However, some individuals may experience allergic reactions or gastrointestinal upset. It may also interact with certain medications or have adverse effects in individuals with certain health conditions. It's important to use agrimony under the guidance of a healthcare professional and to discontinue use if any adverse effects occur.

Alfalfa:

Definition: Alfalfa, scientifically known as Medicago sativa, is a flowering plant in the pea family native to Asia but cultivated worldwide. It's primarily grown as fodder for livestock, but it has also been used in traditional medicine for its potential health benefits.

Ingredients: Alfalfa contains various bioactive compounds, including vitamins (such as vitamin A, vitamin C, and vitamin K), minerals (including calcium, magnesium, and potassium), amino acids, and phytoestrogens. These compounds are believed to contribute to the herb's medicinal properties, including its potential as a nutritive tonic, diuretic, and hormone balancer.

How to Prepare: Alfalfa is typically consumed as sprouts, herbal tea, or in supplement form (such as capsules or tablets). To make tea, dried alfalfa leaves are steeped in hot water for several minutes before being strained and consumed.

Dosage: The appropriate dosage of alfalfa can vary depending on factors such as age, health status, and the specific preparation being used. It's important to follow the recommended dosage on the product label or consult with a qualified herbalist or healthcare professional for personalized guidance.

How to Use: Alfalfa sprouts, tea, or supplements are typically taken orally. It's often consumed as a dietary supplement to support overall health and well-being, as well as to promote kidney health and hormone balance.

Side Effects: Alfalfa is generally considered safe for most people when consumed in moderate amounts. However, some individuals may experience allergic reactions or digestive upset. It may also interact with certain medications or have adverse effects in individuals with certain health conditions, such as autoimmune diseases or hormone-sensitive conditions. Pregnant or breastfeeding individuals should consult with a healthcare professional before using alfalfa supplements. It's important to use alfalfa under the guidance of a healthcare professional and to discontinue use if any adverse effects occur.

Ashwagandha:

Definition: Ashwagandha, scientifically known as Withaniasomnifera, is a small shrub native to India, the Middle East, and parts of Africa. It has a long history of use in Ayurvedic medicine for its potential health benefits, particularly for its adaptogenic properties.

Ingredients: Ashwagandha root contains various bioactive compounds, including alkaloids (such as withanolides), steroidal lactones, and flavonoids. These compounds are believed to contribute to the herb's medicinal properties, including its potential as an adaptogen, anti-inflammatory, and immune-modulating agent.

How to Prepare: Ashwagandha is typically consumed as a powdered root, herbal tea, tincture, or in supplement form (such as capsules or tablets). To make tea, dried ashwagandha root is steeped in hot water for several minutes before being strained and consumed.

Dosage: The appropriate dosage of ashwagandha can vary depending on factors such as age, health status, and the specific preparation being used. It's important to follow the recommended dosage on the product label or consult with a qualified herbalist or healthcare professional for personalized guidance.

How to Use: Ashwagandha powder, tea, tincture, or supplements are typically taken orally. It's often consumed to support stress management, promote relaxation, and boost overall vitality and well-being.

Side Effects: Ashwagandha is generally considered safe for most people when used in moderate amounts. However, some individuals may experience mild side effects such as gastrointestinal upset or drowsiness. It may also interact with certain medications or have adverse effects in individuals with certain health conditions, such as autoimmune diseases or thyroid disorders. Pregnant or breastfeeding individuals should consult with a healthcare professional before using ashwagandha supplements. It's important to use ashwagandha under the guidance of a healthcare professional and to discontinue use if any adverse effects occur.

Astragalus:

Definition: Astragalus, scientifically known as Astragalus membranaceus, is a flowering plant native to China and Mongolia but also found in other parts of Asia. It has been used for centuries in traditional Chinese medicine for its potential health benefits, particularly for its immune-enhancing properties.

Ingredients: Astragalus root contains various bioactive compounds, including polysaccharides, saponins (such as astragalosides), flavonoids, and amino acids. These compounds are believed to contribute to the herb's medicinal properties, including its potential as an adaptogen, immunomodulator, and anti-inflammatory agent.

How to Prepare: Astragalus is typically consumed as a powdered root, herbal tea, tincture, or in supplement form (such as capsules or tablets). To make tea, dried astragalus root slices are simmered in water for several minutes before being strained and consumed.

Dosage: The appropriate dosage of astragalus can vary depending on factors such as age, health status, and the specific preparation being used. It's important to follow the recommended dosage on the product label or consult with a qualified herbalist or healthcare professional for personalized guidance.

How to Use: Astragalus powder, tea, tincture, or supplements are typically taken orally. It's often consumed to support immune function, promote vitality, and enhance overall well-being.

Side Effects: Astragalus is generally considered safe for most people when used in moderate amounts. However, some individuals may experience mild side effects such as gastrointestinal upset or allergic reactions. It may also interact with certain medications or have adverse effects in individuals with certain health conditions, such as autoimmune diseases or diabetes. Pregnant or breastfeeding individuals should consult with a healthcare professional before using astragalus supplements. It's important to use astragalus under the guidance of a healthcare professional and to discontinue use if any adverse effects occur.

Black Cohosh:

Definition: Black cohosh, scientifically known as Actaea racemosa (formerly Cimicifuga racemosa), is a perennial herb native to North America. It has a long history of use in traditional Native American medicine and later in folk medicine for its potential health benefits, particularly for women's health.

Ingredients: Black cohosh root contains various bioactive compounds, including triterpene glycosides (such as actein and cimicifugoside), phenolic acids, and flavonoids. These compounds are believed to contribute to the herb's medicinal properties, including its potential as a hormone-balancing agent and its ability to relieve menopausal symptoms.

How to Prepare: Black cohosh is typically consumed as a powdered root, herbal tea, tincture, or in supplement form (such as capsules or tablets). To make tea, dried black cohosh root is steeped in hot water for several minutes before being strained and consumed.

Dosage: The appropriate dosage of black cohosh can vary depending on factors such as age, health status, and the specific preparation being used. It's important to follow the recommended dosage on the product label or consult with a qualified herbalist or healthcare professional for personalized guidance.

How to Use: Black cohosh powder, tea, tincture, or supplements are typically taken orally. It's often used by women to support hormonal balance, relieve menopausal symptoms such as hot flashes and night sweats, and promote overall well-being.

Side Effects: Black cohosh is generally considered safe for most people when used in moderate amounts. However, some individuals may experience mild side effects such as gastrointestinal upset or allergic reactions. It may also interact with certain medications or have adverse effects in individuals with certain health conditions, such as liver disease or hormone-sensitive conditions. Pregnant or breastfeeding individuals should consult with a healthcare professional before using black cohosh supplements. It's important to use black cohosh under the guidance of a healthcare professional and to discontinue use if any adverse effects occur.

Blessed Thistle:

Definition: Blessed thistle, scientifically known as Cnicusbenedictus, is an annual or biennial herb native to the Mediterranean region but also found in other parts of Europe, Asia, and North Africa. It has been used historically in traditional medicine for its potential health benefits, particularly for digestive and liver health.

Ingredients: Blessed thistle contains various bioactive compounds, including sesquiterpene lactones (such as cnicin), flavonoids, tannins, and essential oils. These compounds are believed to contribute to the herb's medicinal properties, including its potential as a digestive tonic, appetite stimulant, and liver tonic.

How to Prepare: Blessed thistle is typically consumed as an herbal tea, tincture, or in supplement form (such as capsules or tablets). To make tea, dried blessed thistle leaves and flowers are steeped in hot water for several minutes before being strained and consumed.

Dosage: The appropriate dosage of blessed thistle can vary depending on factors such as age, health status, and the specific preparation being used. It's important to follow the recommended dosage on the product label or consult with a qualified herbalist or healthcare professional for personalized guidance.

How to Use: Blessed thistle tea, tincture, or supplements are typically taken orally. It's often used to support digestion, stimulate appetite, and promote liver health.

Side Effects: Blessed thistle is generally considered safe for most people when used in moderate amounts. However, some individuals may experience mild side effects such as gastrointestinal upset or allergic reactions. It may also interact with certain medications or have adverse effects in individuals with certain health conditions, such as hormone-sensitive conditions or bleeding disorders. Pregnant or breastfeeding individuals should consult with a healthcare professional before using blessed thistle supplements. It's important to use blessed thistle under the guidance of a healthcare professional and to discontinue use if any adverse effects occur.

Cat's Claw:

Definition: Cat's claw, scientifically known as Uncaria tomentosa, is a woody vine native to the Amazon rainforest and other parts of Central and South America. It has been used for centuries in traditional medicine by indigenous peoples for its potential health benefits.

Ingredients: Cat's claw contains various bioactive compounds, including alkaloids (such as oxindole alkaloids and quinovic acid glycosides), polyphenols, and other phytochemicals. These compounds are believed to contribute to the herb's medicinal properties, including its potential as an immune enhancer, anti-inflammatory, and antioxidant.

How to Prepare: Cat's claw is typically consumed as an herbal tea, tincture, or in supplement form (such as capsules or tablets). To make tea, dried cat's claw bark or leaves are steeped in hot water for several minutes before being strained and consumed.

Dosage: The appropriate dosage of cat's claw can vary depending on factors such as age, health status, and the specific preparation being used. It's important to follow the recommended dosage on the product label or consult with a qualified herbalist or healthcare professional for personalized guidance.

How to Use: Cat's claw tea, tincture, or supplements are typically taken orally. It's often used to support immune function, reduce inflammation, and promote overall well-being.

Side Effects: Cat's claw is generally considered safe for most people when used in moderate amounts. However, some individuals may experience mild side effects such as gastrointestinal upset or allergic reactions. It may also interact with certain medications or have adverse effects in individuals with certain health conditions, such as autoimmune diseases or bleeding disorders. Pregnant or breastfeeding individuals should consult with a healthcare professional before using cat's claw supplements. It's important to use cat's claw under the guidance of a healthcare professional and to discontinue use if any adverse effects occur.

Chickweed:

Definition: Chickweed, scientifically known as Stellaria media, is an annual herbaceous plant native to Europe but naturalized in many other parts of the world. It's often considered a common weed but has been used historically in traditional medicine for its potential health benefits.

Ingredients: Chickweed contains various bioactive compounds, including flavonoids, saponins, mucilage, and vitamins (such as vitamin C). These compounds are believed to contribute to the herb's medicinal properties, including its potential as a demulcent, anti-inflammatory, and mild diuretic.

How to Prepare: Chickweed is typically consumed as an herbal tea, infusion, or in fresh salads. To make tea, dried chickweed leaves and flowers are steeped in hot water for several minutes before being strained and consumed. It can also be used topically as a poultice or infused oil for skin conditions.

Dosage: The appropriate dosage of chickweed can vary depending on factors such as age, health status, and the specific preparation being used. It's important to follow the recommended dosage on the product label or consult with a qualified herbalist or healthcare professional for personalized guidance.

How to Use: Chickweed tea, infusion, or fresh leaves are typically taken orally. It's often used to soothe inflammation, support digestion, and promote overall well-being. Topically, chickweed can be applied to the skin to alleviate itching, irritation, or minor wounds.

Side Effects: Chickweed is generally considered safe for most people when consumed in moderate amounts. However, some individuals may experience allergic reactions or gastrointestinal upset. It may also interact with certain medications or have adverse effects in individuals with certain health conditions. Pregnant or breastfeeding individuals should consult with a healthcare professional before using chickweed supplements. It's important to use chickweed under the guidance of a healthcare professional and to discontinue use if any adverse effects occur.

Cleavers:

Definition: Cleavers, scientifically known as Galium aparine, is a herbaceous annual plant native to Europe, North America, Asia, and Australia. It has a long history of use in traditional medicine for its potential health benefits.

Ingredients: Cleavers contains various bioactive compounds, including iridoid glycosides, flavonoids, tannins, and mucilage. These compounds are believed to contribute to the herb's medicinal properties, including its potential as a diuretic, lymphatic tonic, and mild astringent.

How to Prepare: Cleavers is typically consumed as an herbal tea, infusion, or in fresh salads. To make tea, dried cleavers leaves and stems are steeped in hot water for several minutes before being strained and consumed. It can also be used topically as a poultice or infused oil for skin conditions.

Dosage: The appropriate dosage of cleavers can vary depending on factors such as age, health status, and the specific preparation being used. It's important to follow the recommended dosage on the product label or consult with a qualified herbalist or healthcare professional for personalized guidance.

How to Use: Cleavers tea, infusion, or fresh leaves are typically taken orally. It's often used to support lymphatic drainage, promote urinary tract health, and soothe inflammation. Topically, cleavers can be applied to the skin to alleviate itching, irritation, or minor wounds.

Side Effects: Cleavers is generally considered safe for most people when consumed in moderate amounts. However, some individuals may experience allergic reactions or gastrointestinal upset. It may also interact with certain medications or have adverse effects in individuals with certain health conditions. Pregnant or breastfeeding individuals should consult with a healthcare professional before using cleavers supplements. It's important to use cleavers under the guidance of a healthcare professional and to discontinue use if any adverse effects occur.

Eucalyptus:

Definition: Eucalyptus refers to a genus of flowering trees and shrubs, primarily native to Australia but also found in other parts of the world. Eucalyptus essential oil, extracted from the leaves of certain species, has a long history of use in traditional medicine for its potential health benefits.

Ingredients: Eucalyptus essential oil contains various bioactive compounds, including eucalyptol (cineole), terpenes, and flavonoids. These compounds are believed to contribute to the oil's medicinal properties, including its potential as an expectorant, decongestant, antiseptic, and anti-inflammatory.

How to Prepare: Eucalyptus essential oil can be used in aromatherapy, diffused in the air, or diluted and applied topically to the skin. It can also be added to steam inhalations or chest rubs to help relieve respiratory symptoms.

Dosage: The appropriate dosage of eucalyptus essential oil can vary depending on factors such as age, health status, and the specific application being used. It's important to follow the recommended dosage on the product label or consult with a qualified aromatherapist or healthcare professional for personalized guidance.

How to Use: Eucalyptus essential oil can be used aromatically, topically, or internally, depending on the intended application. It's often used to alleviate respiratory congestion, soothe sore muscles, promote relaxation, and support overall well-being.

Side Effects: Eucalyptus essential oil is generally considered safe for most people when used appropriately. However, it can be toxic if ingested in large amounts and should not be applied directly to the skin without proper dilution. Some individuals may experience allergic reactions or respiratory irritation when exposed to eucalyptus oil. It's important to use eucalyptus oil with caution, especially around children and pets. Pregnant or breastfeeding individuals should consult with a healthcare professional before using eucalyptus oil. If any adverse effects occur, discontinue use and seek medical attention.

Ginseng:

Definition: Ginseng refers to several species of perennial plants belonging to the Panax genus, including Panax ginseng (Asian ginseng) and Panax quinquefolius (American ginseng). Ginseng has been used for centuries in traditional medicine, particularly in East Asia, for its potential health benefits.

Ingredients: Ginseng root contains various bioactive compounds, including ginsenosides, polysaccharides, and peptides. These compounds are believed to contribute to the herb's medicinal properties, including its potential as an adaptogen, immune enhancer, and cognitive booster.

How to Prepare: Ginseng is typically consumed as a powdered root, herbal tea, tincture, or in supplement form (such as capsules or tablets). To make tea, dried ginseng root slices are simmered in water for several minutes before being strained and consumed.

Dosage: The appropriate dosage of ginseng can vary depending on factors such as age, health status, and the specific preparation being used. It's important to follow the recommended dosage on the product label or consult with a qualified herbalist or healthcare professional for personalized guidance.

How to Use: Ginseng powder, tea, tincture, or supplements are typically taken orally. It's often used to support energy levels, enhance cognitive function, and promote overall well-being.

Side Effects: Ginseng is generally considered safe for most people when used in moderate amounts. However, some individuals may experience mild side effects such as insomnia, gastrointestinal upset, or headaches. It may also interact with certain medications or have adverse effects in individuals with certain health conditions, such as high blood pressure or diabetes. Pregnant or breastfeeding individuals should consult with a healthcare professional before using ginseng supplements. It's important to use ginseng under the guidance of a healthcare professional and to discontinue use if any adverse effects occur.

Goldenseal:

Definition: Goldenseal, scientifically known as Hydrastis canadensis, is a perennial herb native to North America. It has a long history of use in traditional Native American medicine and later in folk medicine for its potential health benefits.

Ingredients: Goldenseal root contains various bioactive compounds, including alkaloids (such as berberine and hydrastine), flavonoids, and volatile oils. These compounds are believed to contribute to the herb's medicinal properties, including its potential as an antimicrobial, anti-inflammatory, and immune enhancer.

How to Prepare: Goldenseal is typically consumed as an herbal tea, tincture, or in supplement form (such as capsules or tablets). To make tea, dried goldenseal root or leaves are steeped in hot water for several minutes before being strained and consumed.

Dosage: The appropriate dosage of goldenseal can vary depending on factors such as age, health status, and the specific preparation being used. It's important to follow the recommended dosage on the product label or consult with a qualified herbalist or healthcare professional for personalized guidance.

How to Use: Goldenseal tea, tincture, or supplements are typically taken orally. It's often used to support immune function, promote digestive health, and soothe inflammation.

Side Effects: Goldenseal is generally considered safe for most people when used in moderate amounts. However, some individuals may experience mild side effects such as gastrointestinal upset or allergic reactions. It may also interact with certain medications or have adverse effects in individuals with certain health conditions, such as high blood pressure or pregnancy. It's important to use goldenseal under the guidance of a healthcare professional and to discontinue use if any adverse effects occur.

Bio Ferro Tonic:

Definition: Bio Ferro Tonic is a dietary supplement primarily composed of herbs and minerals. It's often marketed as a natural way to support overall health, particularly by promoting blood health and circulation.

Ingredients: Typical ingredients in Bio Ferro Tonic may include a blend of herbs such as burdock root, yellow dock root, sarsaparilla root, and cascara sagrada bark, along with minerals like iron and potassium phosphate.

How to Prepare: Bio Ferro Tonic usually comes in liquid form and is typically taken orally. It's important to follow the instructions on the product label for dosage and administration.

Dosage: The dosage can vary depending on the specific product and individual needs. It's crucial to consult with a healthcare professional or follow the recommended dosage on the product label to avoid potential side effects.

How to Use: Bio Ferro Tonic is often taken by adding the recommended dosage to water or juice and consuming it orally. It's important to shake the bottle well before use and store it according to the manufacturer's instructions.

Side Effects: While Bio Ferro Tonic is generally considered safe when used as directed, some individuals may experience side effects such as digestive discomfort, allergic reactions, or interactions with medications. It's essential to consult with a healthcare provider before starting any new supplement regimen, especially if you have underlying health conditions or are taking medications.

Bladderwrack:

Definition: Bladderwrack is a type of seaweed or marine algae commonly used in traditional medicine and as a dietary supplement. It's known for its potential health benefits, particularly related to thyroid health and weight management.

Ingredients: Bladderwrack contains various nutrients, including iodine, vitamins, minerals, and antioxidants. The primary active components are iodine and fucoidan, a type of carbohydrate found in brown seaweeds.

How to Prepare: Bladderwrack supplements are available in various forms, including capsules, powders, and liquid extracts. They can be taken orally with water or added to smoothies and other beverages.

Dosage: The appropriate dosage of bladderwrack can vary based on factors such as age, health status, and the specific product being used. It's essential to follow the recommended dosage on the product label or consult with a healthcare professional for personalized guidance.

How to Use: Bladderwrack supplements are typically taken orally, either with water or mixed into food or beverages. It's important to follow the instructions on the product label and avoid exceeding the recommended dosage.

Side Effects: While bladderwrack is generally considered safe for most people when used in moderation, excessive intake of iodine from bladderwrack supplements can cause thyroid dysfunction and other adverse effects. Individuals with thyroid disorders, iodine sensitivity, or certain medical conditions should exercise caution and consult with a healthcare provider before using bladderwrack supplements. Common side effects may include digestive upset, allergic reactions, or interactions with medications.

Blood Purifier:

Definition: Blood purifiers are herbal remedies or dietary supplements believed to cleanse or detoxify the blood, often promoting overall health and well-being. They are thought to support the body's natural detoxification processes and improve blood circulation.

Ingredients: Blood purifiers may contain a variety of herbs and botanical extracts known for their purported cleansing and detoxifying properties. Common ingredients include burdock root, red clover, dandelion root, and yellow dock root, among others.

How to Prepare: Blood purifiers are typically available in various forms, including capsules, tablets, powders, and liquid extracts. They are usually taken orally with water or juice, following the recommended dosage on the product label.

Dosage: The dosage of blood purifiers can vary depending on the specific product and individual needs. It's important to adhere to the recommended dosage on the product label or consult with a healthcare professional for personalized guidance.

How to Use: Blood purifiers are typically taken orally, either with water or mixed into beverages. They are often used as part of a detoxification regimen or to support overall health and vitality.

Side Effects: While blood purifiers are generally considered safe for most people when used as directed, some individuals may experience side effects such as digestive discomfort, allergic reactions, or interactions with medications. It's important to consult with a healthcare provider before starting any new supplement regimen, especially if you have underlying health conditions or are taking medications.

Hops:

Definition: Hops, scientifically known as Humulus lupulus, is a perennial climbing vine native to Europe, Asia, and North America. It is primarily known for its use in brewing beer but has also been used historically in traditional medicine for its potential health benefits.

Ingredients: Hops flowers contain various bioactive compounds, including bitter acids (such as humulone and lupulone), essential oils, flavonoids, and polyphenols. These compounds are believed to contribute to the herb's medicinal properties, including its potential as a sedative, relaxant, and digestive aid.

How to Prepare: Hops is typically consumed as an herbal tea, tincture, or in supplement form (such as capsules or tablets). To make tea, dried hops flowers are steeped in hot water for several minutes before being strained and consumed.

Dosage: The appropriate dosage of hops can vary depending on factors such as age, health status, and the specific preparation being used. It's important to follow the recommended dosage on the product label or consult with a qualified herbalist or healthcare professional for personalized guidance.

How to Use: Hops tea, tincture, or supplements are typically taken orally. It's often used to promote relaxation, relieve anxiety, and support sleep.

Side Effects: Hops is generally considered safe for most people when used in moderate amounts. However, some individuals may experience mild side effects such as drowsiness, gastrointestinal upset, or allergic reactions. It may also interact with certain medications or have adverse effects in individuals with certain health conditions, such as depression or hormone-sensitive conditions. It's important to use hops under the guidance of a healthcare professional and to discontinue use if any adverse effects occur.

Kelp:

Definition: Kelp refers to several species of large brown algae belonging to the Laminariales order. It is commonly found in underwater forests along rocky coastlines around the world. Kelp has been used for centuries in various cultures, particularly in East Asia, for its nutritional and medicinal properties.

Ingredients: Kelp is rich in various nutrients, including iodine, vitamins (such as vitamin K, vitamin C, and B vitamins), minerals (including calcium, magnesium, and potassium), antioxidants, and fiber. These nutrients are believed to contribute to the seaweed's potential health benefits, including its role in thyroid function, bone health, and immune support.

How to Prepare: Kelp is typically consumed dried, powdered, or in supplement form (such as capsules or tablets). It can also be used in cooking, particularly in soups, salads, and stir-fries. Kelp supplements are available in various forms, including powdered extracts, tablets, and liquid extracts.

Dosage: The appropriate dosage of kelp can vary depending on factors such as age, health status, and the specific preparation being used. It's important to follow the recommended dosage on the product label or consult with a qualified healthcare professional for personalized guidance.

How to Use: Kelp supplements are typically taken orally with water. They can be consumed as part of a daily nutritional regimen to support overall health and well-being. Kelp can also be incorporated into recipes as a flavorful and nutritious ingredient.

Side Effects: While kelp is generally considered safe for most people when consumed in moderate amounts, excessive intake of iodine-rich foods or supplements, including kelp, can lead to thyroid dysfunction or iodine toxicity. Some individuals may also be allergic to seaweed and experience allergic reactions. Pregnant or breastfeeding individuals should consult with a healthcare professional before using kelp supplements. It's important to use kelp under the guidance of a healthcare professional and to discontinue use if any adverse effects occur.

Feverfew:

Definition: Feverfew, scientifically known as Tanacetum parthenium, is a perennial herb native to Europe but also found in other parts of the world. It has a long history of use in traditional medicine, particularly in European folk medicine, for its potential health benefits.

Ingredients: Feverfew contains various bioactive compounds, including sesquiterpene lactones (such as parthenolide), flavonoids, and volatile oils. These compounds are believed to contribute to the herb's medicinal properties, including its potential as an anti-inflammatory, analgesic, and migraine prophylactic.

How to Prepare: Feverfew is typically consumed as an herbal tea, tincture, or in supplement form (such as capsules or tablets). To make tea, dried feverfew leaves and flowers are steeped in hot water for several minutes before being strained and consumed.

Dosage: The appropriate dosage of feverfew can vary depending on factors such as age, health status, and the specific preparation being used. It's important to follow the recommended dosage on the product label or consult with a qualified herbalist or healthcare professional for personalized guidance.

How to Use: Feverfew tea, tincture, or supplements are typically taken orally. It's often used to alleviate headaches, including migraines, and to support overall well-being.

Side Effects: Feverfew is generally considered safe for most people when used in moderate amounts. However, some individuals may experience mild side effects such as gastrointestinal upset or allergic reactions. It may also interact with certain medications or have adverse effects in individuals with certain health conditions, such as bleeding disorders or pregnancy. It's important to use feverfew under the guidance of a healthcare professional and to discontinue use if any adverse effects occur.

THE END